Sugar Detox

Sugar Detox for Beginners,
Including a 30 Day Meal Plan,
Energy Boosting Recipes,
And Tips on Staying Sugar Free

by
Josh West

Table of Contents

Introduction

I want to thank you for buying the book Sugar Detox: Sugar Detox for Beginners - Including a 30 Day Meal Plan, Energy Boosting Recipes, and Tips on Staying Sugar Free.

This book contains proven steps and strategies on how to become a truly healthier person by learning the effects sugar has on the human body and applying this knowledge to day-to-day life.

"Sugar Detox" not only supplies the necessary tools to get started on the path to a healthier lifestyle, this book provides the insight as to how and why while listing delicious recipes, a thirty day detox diet, and what life is like without unhealthy amounts of sugar.

Here is an inescapable fact: you will need to understand that willpower is a way of getting your mind around a biological process.

In a world plagued with crash diets, dangerous detoxes, and diet pill fads that only cater to instant gratification, this book shines a light on how educating yourself and applying that knowledge in everyday life leads to a much healthier lifestyle; mind, body, and spirit.

It's science, but it's not rocket science. When deciding to lose weight or make healthier choices in eating habits, getting started can be daunting. In the mind, it could equivocate to being too complex, difficult, or something that will just never be grasped.

Take this molecular formula for example: $C_{12}H_{22}O_{11}$. For those of us who do not wear a lab coat to work, that formula is sucrose, commonly known as sugar. Sugar Detox calls it like it is in terms that are easily understood, with no guess work, confusing formulas, or conflicting ideology, and is based on proven facts.

If you do not develop your understanding of how your own body works and what it needs to function well, the consequences can be vast and long-lasting, and in some cases irreversible. Would you like more lasting energy, fewer cravings, reduced body fat, a more balanced temperament, and/or clearer thinking? Sugar Detox offers a helpful, no nonsense approach to resolving these issues and more.

It's time for you to become an amazing champion of sugar detoxing by simply putting to practice what you will learn in this book. The information contained in this book will change your life. You will become more informed about the inner workings of your own body and it will benefit you in ways that will be long lasting and long reaching.

The genius in the simplicity of Sugar Detox is that it's right in front of you. Have you ever misplaced your glasses or sunglasses, frantically searching high and low to no avail, only to discover that they have been on your head the entire time? It is the same with a sugar detox. It is within your reach, you only needed to discover it for yourself.

Welcome to Sugar Detox!

Chapter 1. How We Become Addicted to Sugar

Most people enjoy rewarding themselves from time to time. From having a beer after work on payday to a late night slice of chocolate layered cake after a stressful day, it just feels good. Right? Right!

The reason we enjoy these things and why it can easily turn into an addiction is purely biological. It is a reward system. This system is a series of chemical and electrical path systems across different areas of the brain.

When foods are consumed that have a high sugar content, the brain is bombarded with dopamine, a neurotransmitter that talks to the brain and tells us that sugar makes us feel good. The human brain has many dopamine receptors.

When foods high in sugar are consumed frequently and in large amounts, fewer receptors become available to absorb the dopamine, which results in lower levels of dopamine.

Less dopamine means that the same amount of sugar just will not cut it. This in turn leads to higher consumption of sugar in order to get the same feel-good feeling and it all very quickly and ultimately becomes a giant catch twenty two.

Sugar has officially and undeniably hijacked your brain.

Sugar also triggers the hormone serotonin, a calming hormone in the brain. Since sugar and other junk foods have such a drastic effect on the reward centers of the brain, the result is very similar to that of abused drugs like heroin, cocaine, nicotine and marijuana.

The exact same brain centers are at work here. (The slang term "dope" to describe illegal drugs actually derives from the word dopamine, because of the effect it has on the brain.)

This fact can be really unnerving, considering that an extremely high amount of sugar in one form or another is found in so many foods and beverages that we consume on a daily basis, with consistency.

How often do we hear of drug addicts constantly in and out of rehab? How many products are there on the market for people who are addicted to nicotine? Have you ever heard of sugar-holics anonymous? The idea seems preposterous, but the effects on the brain are the same and equally important to understand.

The effects on the body are less severe, but detrimental nonetheless. People who have a certain predisposition toward addiction become highly addicted to these high sugar foods and drinks, ultimately losing control over their consumption of these items, resulting in strong addition, obesity and other dangerous side effects.

Basically this is how sugar and junk food hijack the brain chemistry to make us crave more and eat more and crave more and eat more and so on.

In some cases, people will experience actual anatomical changes to the brain when exposed to a diet high in sugar. The brain physically changes. In most of these cases, the person becomes highly addicted.

Addiction to sugar is exactly the same as being addicted to nicotine, marijuana, and narcotics. For reiteration purposes, the brain reacts exactly the same way to high doses of sugar as it does to illegal drugs!

There is no difference aside from the substance being abused and the consequences of a relapse with sugar are less serious. Substance abuse researchers performed brain scans on people who had consumed sugar. Their results reflected that when test subjects consume sugar, the parts of the brain that light up are the same parts as an alcoholic with a bottle of booze.

Chapter 2. Reasons to Reduce Our Sugar Intake

Aside from unhealthy addiction, there is an extremely long list of reasons t0 reduce your sugar intake. These reasons range from unhealthy brain function to mood alteration to obesity to avoiding cancer.

Researchers' studies have shown that too much sugar actually impairs brain function, causes liver damage and obesity, wreaks havoc on our metabolism, and could leave us susceptible to diabetes, heart disease, and even cancer.

Unfortunately with about 80% of our available food containing sugar, it is difficult to avoid consuming unhealthy amounts.

How Sugar Affects the Brain and Nervous System

Some studies have suggested that sugar forms free radicals in the brain's membrane which undermines the nerve cells' ability to effectively communicate. This could affect how well instructions are remembered, ideas are processed, and moods are handled. This can make you seem like a "different person" to those who may know you.

As stated earlier in Sugar Detox, refined sugar is a carbohydrate. In particular it is a carbohydrate that our bodies are not built to metabolize, especially in large quantities.

Incomplete metabolism of carbohydrates results in forming what is known as toxic metabolites, such as pyruvic acid.

Pyruvic acid collects in red blood cells, the brain, and the nervous system. The toxic metabolites then interfere with the cells' ability to 'breathe', meaning that the cells are unable to receive enough oxygen to survive and function normally.

Over time, some of these cells completely die off, which ultimately leads to the beginning of degenerative disease. Sugar also promotes depression.

After a 6 year study of 9,000 test subjects, it was discovered that those who consumed the most sugar were nearly 40% more at risk of depression than those who did not partake in high amounts of the sweet stuff. Bummer.

How Sugar Affects the Skin

Simple carbohydrates such as white bread, refined sugar, and soft drinks, cause insulin levels to spike. This spike in insulin results in a sudden inflammation of the body.

This sudden inflammation produces enzymes that break down elastin and collagen. Collagen and elastin are proteins in the skin which keep the skin elastic and firm.

When these proteins are attacked by enzymes, the results are sagging skin and wrinkles. Yes, sugar causes you to age more quickly. Not only that, but the sagging and wrinkles are now irreversible.

In addition to increasing the effects of aging, refined sugar also exacerbates preexisting skin conditions such as acne, psoriasis, and eczema. The more sugar you consume, the more likely you are to develop an insulin resistance.

Insulin resistance may manifest as dark patches on the skin in the neck area and in body creases such as the armpits. Insulin resistance can also lead to dull looking skin and rapid hair growth – usually in extremely unwanted areas.

Sugar also dehydrates your skin cells, causing redness, puffiness, and circles under the eyes.

The Role of Sugar in Tooth Decay

Poor oral health and sugar consumption go hand in hand. Plaque is constantly forming on your teeth and gums. Plaque contains bacteria which feeds on the sugars you ingest, creating enamel eating acids that start to eat away at your teeth as soon as within 20 seconds of contact.

After the acid eats through even the tiniest microscopic part of the enamel, it starts eating away at the rest of the tooth, causing cavities and tooth rot. Sugar literally rots your teeth.

The amount of sugar consumed at one time has less negative impact on your tooth enamel than how consistently you consume sugar. If you chug a soda, your tooth enamel has more chance of surviving than if you sipped a soda over the course of an hour, because the acids have a shorter window to do their damage.

Of course, it wouldn't be such a bad idea to completely eliminate soft drinks from your diet altogether. Why tempt fate? Erosion of tooth enamel can lead to much more serious consequences than just a cavity. Serious erosion can lead to:

- A significant wearing down of your back molars – these are the teeth that primarily allow us to chew our food, whether you're a vegetarian or not. Imagine you're on a fancy dinner date, trying desperately to politely and gracefully chew your food without any back molars. Mashed potatoes please!

- Tooth loss and extraction of unhealthy teeth – it is an extremely slippery slope. Since teeth are in such close proximity to each other and in less than sterile living conditions, if one gets "sick", the more likely it is for the teeth on either side to get sick too.

- Extreme changes to your bite – your bite is the way your upper and lower teeth come together. This affects your smile and how effectively you are able to chew your food, which it also affects your digestion.

- Having to replace damaged dental work – fillings and other dental work have been known to fall out or corrode from the teeth not being cared for properly. Not only can this cause excruciating pain, it also adds to the inconvenience of taking up time and money.

- Dental implants – if you're lucky enough to be able to afford dental implants, that is. They are highly costly and cause a great deal of pain for a considerable amount of time.

- Gum surgery – surgery. In your mouth. The reason mouth pain tends to be so severe is not only because your teeth are directly connected to nerve endings, but also the mouth is full of all kinds of bacteria that can make the healing process seem like it will never end.

Sugar and the Body in General

The average American consumes approximately 130 pounds of *added* sugar each year. Keep in mind that this statistic includes only added sugar, not sugar that is already naturally occurring, as in fruit or milk.

Sugar adds fatty tissue to your organs, essentially making your organs 'fat'. Added sugars trigger your liver into storing fat in odd places, and the liver does this so very efficiently.

As odd as this may sound, your liver hiding Easter eggs of fat within itself leads to liver disease, a thing rarely seen before 1980 but has unfortunately has since become a common occurrence.

A study published in the Journal of the American Medical Association found that those test subjects who consumed the highest amounts of added sugar also showed the biggest spike in bad cholesterol levels and harmful triglyceride blood fats, as well as exhibiting the lowest dip in good cholesterol levels.

One theory is that sugar overload sparks your liver to churn out higher levels of bad cholesterol, while simultaneously inhibiting the liver's ability to effectively clear it out.

Added sugars also cause high amounts of insulin to be released into the arteries. Consistently high insulin levels cause the muscle cells surrounding each blood vessel to grow much more rapidly than normal.

This results in hard arterial walls, which then leads to high blood pressure and makes a heart attack or stroke that much more likely.

High amounts of sugar decrease the hormone leptin's ability to tell your body that it has had enough food, effectively leading to consistent overeating.

Sugar is also proven to starve your body of energy. After a short microburst of energy, the body goes from sugar rush to sugar crash, because when sugar hits the brain, it triggers the release of serotonin, a sleep regulator.

Chapter 3. The Health Benefits of a Sugar Detox

The benefits of choosing to sugar detox are all as interconnected as they are numerous. Hence the following benefits are in no particular order of importance, because they are all spectacularly well worth it.

- Clearer thinking – you'll get your brain back! You'll be able to think more clearly, reason more cognitively and compute more efficiently. Just as importantly, you'll forever be rid of those sugar induced mood swings!

- Increased stamina – you'll have more energy and longer lasting energy, which in and of itself opens up a whole new world of possibilities. What could you accomplish with more energy every day? Exciting!

- Healthier sleeping habits – with your body not constantly being bombarded by serotonin, the brain will naturally revert to a healthy reaction to serotonin. Instead of waving it off as yet another pest beating down its door, the brain will welcome the serotonin with open arms, resulting in more restful sleep.

- Weight loss – you will absolutely lose weight on this detox, but the point is to provide you with the tools necessary to make healthier eating choices, which will naturally result in a more svelte physique.

- Save money – making more healthful choices in your diet will lead to fewer health issues, which leads to saving your hard earned money for more enjoyable things than costly medical bills.

- Better skin – you'll enjoy healthy, glowing skin, fewer wrinkles, and less sagging. You will look and feel better, and it will show to everyone around you.

- A stronger connection with your inner self – instead of wasting time and energy worrying about things that are out of your control in life, you will be focused on a solid goal. How you relate to the world will make you happier and feel more at peace. You will feel more comfortable in your own healthy new skin, which will inspire and uplift the people with whom you come in contact.

Chapter 4. Foods and Beverages to Avoid

Added sugar

Avoid ALL *added* sugar – artificial or otherwise, no exceptions. This is a fairly challenging endeavor as most sugar goes by many different names.

Note that the following list is not exhaustive, but it does include most of the forms of sugar that you would most likely come across in an everyday situation.

It is *far* too easy to be tricked into eating something that has sugar in it, and an extremely high amount of sugar even. The following added sugars to avoid are placed in alphabetical order for ease of reference.

- Agave nectar/syrup, aspartame, barley malt, beet sugar, cane juice, cane sugar, confectioner's sugar, corn sugar, corn sweetener, corn syrup, corn syrup solids, crystallized fructose, date sugar, dextran, dextrose, evaporated cane juice, fructose, fruit juice, fruit juice concentrate, glucose, glucose solids, glucose sugar, grape juice concentrate, grape sugar, honey, invert sugar, lactose, malt, maltodextrin, maltose, mannitol, molasses, polydextrose, raw sugar, saccharin, sorghum, sucralose, sucrose, stevia, sugar (of course), syrup (all), turbinado sugar, xylitol, and zeroes

Additives

- MSG, trans fat; also foods like ketchup, salad dressings, salsas, and spaghetti sauce

All whole fruits, with the exception of lemon and lime only

Starches and grains

- Bran, bread, buckwheat, cereal, corn products (there are *so* many of them!), cracked barley, germ, granola, millet, oatmeal, oats, tortillas, and white rice

Others

- Alcohol – all forms
- Candy
- Chocolate
- Dairy – all forms (until later in the detox)
- Desserts
- Fast food
- Fried food
- Juices, especially ones made from concentrate
- Legumes
- Prepackaged drinks and food
- Processed foods
- Pizza
- Soft drinks
- White bread

Foods and Beverages that Adhere to the Sugar Detox Standards

- Avocado
- Beef (free range, grass fed)
- Berries (on and after day 15)
- Bone broth
- Brown rice
- Chocolate (*strictly* 100% unsweetened only! No exceptions!)
- Chicken (free range)
- Cider
- Coconut milk
- Coconut oil
- Eggs
- Fish (fresh only)
- Ghee
- Grape seed oil
- Green beans (very small amounts)
- Herbal tea
- Kombucha (on and after day 3 and *highly* recommended once per day to help curb sugar cravings – it works!)
- Lamb (free range)
- Leafy greens
- Lemon
- Lime
- Nut butters (no sugar added only, and no cashew butter)
- Nuts (with the exception of cashews)
- Olive oil (in all of its forms)

- Pork (free range)
- Quinoa
- Seaweed
- Seeds
- Smoothies
- Tomatoes
- Turkey (free range)
- Vanilla (only from vanilla pod)
- Vegetables
- Vinegars
- Water (of course. If you get bored with your water try freezing herbs like rosemary or cilantro in your ice cubes and try a squeeze of lemon or lime)
- Whole fruits (on and after day 15)
- Whole grains (on and after day 15)

Keep in mind that while great pains have been taken to compile these lists, if you have any questions, use your best judgment or consult someone who will be able to answer your questions like a nutritionist or a blogger educated on and well versed in, sugar detox.

Chapter 5. Preparing for Your Sugar Detox

Set yourself up for success! In order to participate in and ultimately succeed in a sugar detox, you must adequately prepare yourself for what lies ahead. You are about to embark on an amazing betterment of yourself and it will only behoove you to plan accordingly. Here are a few steps to take in order to achieve your goals and ensure that it is as easy as possible.

1. **Detox your home –**

    Get rid of ALL of the things in your refrigerator, freezer, cupboards, pantry, etc. that don't fit in with the sugar detox. If you find it difficult to get rid of your old familiar favorites, you are not alone. However, as difficult as this may be, it is absolutely crucial that you are not swayed by temptation, especially early on.

    It is completely understandable to not want to waste perfectly good food. You do have two options here. You can plan far enough ahead to consume your favorite foods, leftovers and open containers. You can simply give the food away to an appreciative neighbor, friend, or family member. You can also do a combination of these things but just make sure that ALL of the foods, beverages, etc. that need to be avoided are out of the house – for good.

2. **Gather what you need –**

Go grocery shopping. Write out your grocery list and make sure that you get ONLY those items allowed for the sugar detox diet. It is imperative that the first grocery shopping trip should only include those items you will need for the **first three days**.

This can be vital to success, since the first three days require a much more strict diet than the rest of the meal plan. Check and recheck this list. On the third day, make up another list and shop for items that are allowed for the sugar detox diet **up until day 14**, again making doubly sure that only items that are allowed from days 1 to 14 make their way into your house.

Repeat this process on day 14 to shop for the rest of the items you will need for the remainder of the detox. This will be made much easier by the fact that at that time you will have developed a craving for less sugary, processed foods and will have become accustomed to this new diet.

3. **Taper off caffeine, alcohol, and sugar –**

The length of time you spend on tapering off depends entirely on the amounts of which you consume these items, and the frequency.

Avid coffee drinker? Enjoy a couple of drinks after work a few times a week? Constantly consuming soft drinks, other drinks high in sugar, or treating yourself to sweets?

You may want to start tapering off **at least** two weeks and up to a month ahead of your planned start date. If you enjoy caffeine, alcohol, and sugar moderately, you may want to start tapering off at least one week before the day you plan to start the sugar detox.

This is a very necessary step in the process of preparing for a sugar detox for a couple of reasons.

It's much healthier than quitting cold turkey. Your body may go through unhealthy withdrawals if you consume caffeine, alcohol, and sugar in excess, and then just stop altogether.

Psychologically speaking, tapering off puts your will power and thinking in the right frame of mind. This is like starting a race with your toe at the starting line, as opposed to just ogling the race track on the sidelines.

4. **Align your intentions and your mind –**

This is why it is so important to taper off your intake of caffeine, alcohol, and sugar. If your mind and body don't physically need these things as much as it used to, the mind becomes much more receptive to further change.

This process is the equivalent of starting to set rules and boundaries for a child who has never or rarely been told, "No". If this is done slowly, steadily, and with great care, the end result is infinitely more successful and rewarding than if this were to happen suddenly and harshly.

Set goals. Think about what day one on the sugar detox will be like and think positively. This is an exciting adventure, and if you align your mind and intentions along those lines (or whatever may work best for you) your adventure will be much more successful and rewarding than if you had not.

If you start thinking begrudgingly about the sugar detox before you even have a chance to begin, you are pretty much setting yourself up for failure. It is human nature to be scared of and to resent change, so if you find yourself thinking about the sugar detox in a negative light, follow that negative thought immediately with a positive thought. For example: "Ugh, I can't believe I am putting myself through this. What was I thinking?!"

That negative thought should immediately be followed up by a positive thought like, "But I have the power to do this and it will be something different and rewarding, maybe even fun…maybe my friend (so and so) would be interested in this sugar detox so I don't have to do it alone."

It may sound silly, but whatever it takes for you to get your mind and intentions set on your goal, the easier and more successful you will be.

5. **Measure yourself –**

If you do not currently own a body measurement tape and do not know anyone who could lend you one, they are sold pretty much anywhere you could find a sewing kit; grocery stores, drug stores, and super stores just to name a few.

The point of taking your body measurements before you start the sugar detox is so that you can physically track your progress, as well as your end result.

If you measure your waist on week two of the sugar detox and find that you've lost an inch since the last time you measured, your brain accepts this fact as proof that what you're doing is working and that you should continue.

Also, imaging that rewarding day when you've completed the sugar detox successfully and you take all of your measurements again.

Comparing notes with your measurements of when you first started will let you know that you succeeded in accomplishing a difficult goal and will work as testimony of your success for yourself, but those around you.

6. **Start a sugar detox journal –**

You may be thinking that keeping a journal isn't exactly your idea of fun, but it's the only way to document your journey.

What you choose to write is up to you, as is the frequency of which you do it. As a suggestion, start with your measurements before you start the detox. You may choose to document every detail of every day, or you just may include your shopping list and measurement for the week. Aside from taking body measurements on a weekly basis, it is a way for your mind to check in with what is going on with your body. In a sense, that is one way to wrap your brain around what is going on. You will read the journal as you progress, and it will be easier to take the next step and keep on going because your brain will have another source of a visual. Another added benefit of keeping a sugar detox journal is that you can write about any stress or anything you may have overcome and have it to read for yourself or to share with someone you care about. Participating in the sugar detox diet may be emotional for some at one point or another, especially if that person is not detoxing with someone else, and having a journal as an outlet is very healthy - and that is the whole point of starting this detox in the first place – the added health benefits.

Chapter 6. First 3 Day Meal Plan and Recipes

The first three days of the sugar detox eliminates sugar in all of its forms from your diet. This includes sucrose, glucose, fructose, lactose, artificial sweeteners, and other sugars and no carbohydrates.

The good news is it gets easier from there by slowly reintroducing healthier sugar options back into your everyday meals, snacks and beverages.

This may include whole grains, fruits, dairy products, and even a glass of wine or beer. This detox is completely doable as it is not based on depriving yourself of nourishing, delicious foods and beverages you love.

Instead it is solely concentrated on cutting back on and learning how to eliminate the unhealthy amounts of sugars from your diet.

Keep in mind that the sugar detox utilizes the properties of a high protein diet, as well as foods that contain "good" fatty foods such as avocado.

These foods are proven to reduce your body's cravings for sugar, while providing the much needed sustenance and nourishment your body needs.

Set your mind at ease if you are not used to consuming large amounts of these foods, they are absolutely necessary and your body will know exactly what to do with them.

If you happen to be a vegetarian, please feel free to substitute as you see fit, within the guidelines of the sugar detox diet.

Seeing as the first three days of the sugar detox will be the strictest, it is important that the guidelines for these first three days be followed as closely as possible, if not to the letter.

Around the fourth day, you may start experiencing the withdrawal symptoms of eliminating sugar from your diet. These symptoms may include headaches, nervousness, irritability, nausea, and varying degrees of sugar cravings.

The sugar cravings may range anywhere from mild to severe, dependent on how much and how often you consumed high amounts of added sugar and much time you gave yourself to taper off of sugar before you began the detox.

If you find yourself experiencing strong cravings or intense cravings, don't be wary of reaching out to the people in your life that you trust. You can also use the internet to research specific questions or to post on a sugar detox blog.

The people who write these blogs have a lot of insight into what you will be going through and are normally very responsive and extremely supportive.

DAY 1

Breakfast: Spinach baked eggs

For one serving you will need: 1 egg, 1 cup fresh spinach, ramekin or muffin pan.

Cook spinach 5 minutes, then drain. Add drained spinach to bottom of ramekin or muffin pan. Crack one egg on top. Bake for 15 minutes for a runny yolk. Add a few minutes for a firmer yolk. Let cool 5 minutes and serve!

Mid-morning Snack: Baked almonds

For two servings you will need: 1 cookie sheet, ½ cup unsalted almonds, 1 TBSP Bragg's Liquid Aminos. This is a great alternative to soy sauce or table salt. It tastes great and is great for you.

Preheat oven to 350 degrees. Line baking sheet with foil. Toss almonds with liquid aminos. Bake for 5 minutes. Remove from oven and let cool on parchment paper. This snack will keep in an airtight container for one week.

Lunch: Mixed green salad with liquid amino pepper dressing

Per one cup of mixed greens, add 1 tsp of liquid aminos and pepper to taste.

Afternoon snack: 3 hardboiled eggs with yolks removed

Dinner: Baked stuffed chicken with spinach, tomato and cucumber salad

For one serving you will need: Baking dish, 1 chicken breast, ½ cup cooked and spinach, salt, pepper, pinch of rosemary, ½ cucumber and 1 whole tomato.

Preheat oven to 375 degrees. Slice chicken breast in half lengthwise without cutting completely through. In a bowl combine spinach, salt and pepper to taste. Stuff chicken with spinach. Add pinch of rosemary atop chicken. Bake for 35 minutes.

For the salad, coarsely chop cucumber and tomato, adding just a hint of salt to bring out the flavor.

Recommended Beverages for First 3 Days: Water, plain herbal tea

DAY 2

Breakfast: Peanut butter smoothie

For one serving you will need: Blender, 1 ½ tbsp. unsweetened peanut butter, 3/4 cup sugar free almond milk, 1 cup of ice

Combine all ingredients in blender until smooth. Pour into glass and top with an optional unsweetened peanut butter drizzle.

Midmorning Snack: 3 hardboiled eggs with yolk removed

Lunch: Light vegetable soup

You will need: Large sauce pan, 2 tbsp. olive oil, 2 large cloves of garlic - minced, 1 cup chopped onion, 2 cups chopped celery, 4 cups water, 2 cups low sodium vegetable stock or chicken broth, 2 cups fresh spinach – chopped, 1 cup green beans – frozen, ½ tsp salt. ¼ tsp pepper

In a large saucepan, heat oil at medium heat. Then add garlic and cook until aromatic. Add celery and onion. Sauté until veggies get tender, or approximately 10 minutes. Add broth and water and bring to a boil. When boiling, add green beans, salt and pepper. Cover and simmer on low for 30 minutes. Uncover and add spinach. Cook until wilted, approximately 5 minutes.

Afternoon Snack: Left over baked almonds

Dinner: Turkey lettuce wraps

You will need: Saucepan, 2 tbsp. sesame oil, 1 lb. ground turkey, 1 tbsp. fresh minced ginger, ½ cup sliced mushroom, 1 red bell pepper, ½ cup water, ¼ tsp garlic powder, ¼ tsp ground cinnamon, ¼ tsp Emeril's Asian Essence Powder, ½ tsp salt, romaine or Bibb lettuce, ¼ cup chopped cilantro or basil, ½ tsp sesame seeds

Heat oil over medium heat. Add ginger and turkey. After browning turkey, add water, mushrooms and diced pepper and cook until completely heated through. Add cinnamon, garlic powder and salt and heat for 1 to 2 more minutes. Serve mixture onto a single leaf of your choice of greens. Top with your choice of chopped herbs and sesame seeds.

DAY 3

Breakfast: Scrambled eggs with spinach and mushroom, topped with no sugar added salsa

You will need: Skillet or frying pan, 1 tbsp. EVOO, 2 eggs, ¼ cup cooked spinach, ¼ cup sliced mushrooms.

Heat oil on medium heat. In a bowl, combine eggs, spinach, mushrooms, salt and pepper and beat until thoroughly mixed. Pour mixture into pan and cook until eggs are firm, stirring every few seconds. Top with no sugar added salsa.

Midmorning Snack: Baked almonds – see recipe on Day 1

Lunch: Leftover turkey lettuce wraps

Afternoon Snack: Raw veggies (NO CARROTS) with hummus dip.

Dinner: Grilled chicken and fresh herbs, cucumber and tomato salad

You will need: Grill, food processor or high-powered blender, 3 skinless/boneless chicken breasts – sliced lengthwise, 1 cup loosely packed herbs – cilantro, basil and parsley, ¼ cup olive oil, 2 tbsp. Bragg's Liquid Aminos, 2 large garlic cloves, ¼ tsp pepper, 2 tsp salt

Place washed, chopped herbs in food processor or high powered blender. Add liquid aminos, oil, salt, pepper, and garlic. Puree until mixture is smooth. Place chicken and mixture in zip lock bag and massage chicken and marinade for 5 minutes. Marinade for about 3o minutes, or up to 4 hours. Grill chicken 10 – 15 minutes per side, until middle is no longer pink.

Congratulations! You have made it through the first three days of the sugar detox diet, the most difficult part of this journey. Now it's time to slowly start reintroducing fruit, dairy and whole grains.

Chapter 7. 30 Day Meal Plan

DAY 4

Breakfast: Fried egg, avocado half, 2 turkey sausage links, ¼ cup sautéed zucchini

Snack: One stick of string cheese

Lunch: Salad with roasted potatoes

Snack: Fresh veggies with no sugar added peanut butter

Dinner: Lemon-roasted cod, roasted turnips, and Brussel sprouts with pesto

DAY 5

Breakfast: Eggs baked in avocado halves and tomato slices, both topped with basil and goat cheese

Snack: One stick of string cheese

Lunch: Butter lettuce salad with Portobello and shaved almonds, sugar free vinaigrette dressing

Snack: 1 piece of whole fruit

Dinner: Spicy butternut squash and sweet potato soup, your choice of fish steak with lemon

DAY 6

Breakfast: Breakfast salad with spinach, kale, boiled egg, Canadian bacon and half an avocado with juice of half a lemon

Snack: Apple, cottage cheese

Lunch: Whole roasted wild salmon with lemon, capers and kale

Snack: ½ cup raw nuts

Dinner: Spicy Thai pork salad (Thai nom sod)

DAY 7

Breakfast: Fried egg over roasted cauliflower, bacon, and potato hash

Snack: 1 stick string cheese

Lunch: Tomato and white bean salad with oven roasted squash and pesto

Snack: Kale chips

Dinner: Tomato, basil and mushroom meat sauce over whole grain penne pasta

DAY 8

Breakfast: Fried egg, charred cauliflower with almonds and shishito peppers, half an orange

Snack: Brussels sprouts chips

Lunch: Beef stir fry with peppers and onions

Snack: Green fries

Dinner: Chimichurri chicken lettuce cups

DAY 9

Breakfast: Shukshuka

Snack: Apple chips

Lunch: Steamed clams with lemon

Snack: Raw carrots, no sugar added peanut butter and cinnamon

Dinner: Seared scallops over marinated mushrooms and red sorrel

DAY 10

Breakfast: Ham and egg, hash browns, sautéed kale, walnut and radish salad

Snack: Sautéed apple in coconut oil with cinnamon

Lunch: Steamed oysters with lemon

Snack: Baked chili sweet potato chips

Dinner: Sautéed Swiss chard with shitake mushrooms

DAY 11

Breakfast: Smoked wild salmon with capers, lime, and plain yogurt

Snack: Fresh veggies and hummus

Lunch: Hot sausage, carrot mash and leeks

Snack: Bacon guacamole with sweet potato chips

Dinner: Lemon ginger roasted chicken with thyme or rosemary

DAY 12

Breakfast: Savory grain free herb muffins

Snack: Olives and hummus

Lunch: Mixed green salad with mango and chili

Snack: Baked plantain chips with mojo sauce

Dinner: Kale – Azorean soup

DAY 13

Breakfast: Spicy salmon frittata

Snack: 1 granny smith apple

Lunch: Slow roasted herb roast beef

Snack: tomato and basil topped with cottage cheese

Dinner: Seared scallops on top of spinach/ mint/ chickpea puree, roasted mushrooms and mixed veggies

DAY 14

Breakfast: Blueberry coconut baked steel cut oatmeal

Snack: 1 stick of string cheese

Lunch: Homemade bone broth

Snack: Cucumber tomato salad with dill and squeeze of lime

Dinner: Mixed greens salad with cucumber, carrot and apple, homemade raspberry vinaigrette

DAY 15

Breakfast: Vegetable and quinoa breakfast bowl

Snack: Apple and radish salad with dill

Lunch: Homemade chicken soup

Snack: Vegetarian summer roll

Dinner: Chicken with creamy mushroom sauce on a bed of steamed spinach

DAY 16

Breakfast: Fried eggs with avocado and charred tomato

Snack: 1 sliced granny smith apple with no sugar added peanut butter

Lunch: Kale leaf salad

Snack: Lemon deviled eggs, no mayo or mustard

Dinner: Roasted carrot and kale salad with fresh dill

DAY 17

Breakfast: Chia seed breakfast bowl with banana

Snack: 1 peeled orange

Lunch: Brown rice with kale and veggies

Snack: Sweet potato chips with cottage cheese

Dinner: Mixed greens salad with turkey, beets, delicate squash, radish, and pomegranate

DAY 18

Breakfast: Sausage pizza egg muffins

Snack: Cinnamon fruit kabobs

Lunch: Pan roasted chicken thighs with lemon and sage

Snack: Kale chips with squeeze of lemon

Dinner: Creamy tomato and quinoa soup

DAY 19

Breakfast: Eggs baked in prosciutto filled portabella caps

Snack: Sesame roasted carrots

Lunch: Baby spinach and beet salad

Snack: Dilled green beans

Dinner: Micro green salad with hardboiled egg

DAY 20

Breakfast: Soft boiled eggs, sweet potato hash, turkey sausage links

Snack: Quinoa salad

Lunch: Pork adobo

Snack: Fresh veggies with hummus

Dinner: Mixed greens salad with bacon, apple, beets and sweet potato

DAY 21

Breakfast: Mexican omelet with no sugar added salsa

Snack: 1 peach

Lunch: Carrot and cabbage confetti salad

Snack: Kale chips

Dinner: Pork chop, cinnamon applesauce, asparagus

DAY 22

Breakfast: Chicken scotch eggs

Snack: 1 granny smith apple

Lunch: Grilled zucchini and peppers salad

Snack: Steamed broccoli with Kalamata olives

Dinner: Baked stuffed pepper of choice, with chicken, black beans, cottage cheese

DAY 23

Breakfast: Scrambled eggs with fresh veggies, turkey sausage

Snack: Chili roasted pumpkin seeds

Lunch: Roasted carrots with avocado and basil

Snack: Pineapple chicken skewer

Dinner: Chicken con crema, mixed greens salad with strawberries

DAY 24

Breakfast: Spicy avocado egg salad, bacon

Snack: 1 pear

Lunch: Open faced scuttlebutt sandwich on cauliflower bread

Snack: Lettuce wrap sliders

Dinner: Crock pot chicken and bean stew

DAY 25

Breakfast: Southwest shrimp cakes

Snack: Mixed berries

Lunch: Mixed green salad with veggies, beets, and peeled orange slices

Snack: Red curry shrimp skewer with basil and coconut

Dinner: Cornish game hen, roasted sweet potatoes, roasted Brussels sprouts

DAY 26

Breakfast: Green chile salmon muffins, roasted broccoli

Snack: Small slice of cantaloupe with cottage cheese

Lunch: Spicy sausage, arugula and almond salad

Snack: Kale chips

Dinner: Small filet mignon, whole steamed artichoke with creamy lemon pepper/bacon dipping sauce

DAY 27

Breakfast: Bacon butternut squash soup, fried egg

Snack: 1 banana, optional no sugar added peanut butter

Lunch: Roasted chicken, dill beets with mint

Snack: Portabella pizza

Dinner: Coconut curry chicken, roasted cauliflower

DAY 28

Breakfast: Spinach and sausage breakfast casserole

Snack: Fruit salad with squeeze of lemon

Lunch: Kale and micro greens salad with fresh corn and squeeze of lemon

Snack: Veggies and summer squash hummus

Dinner: Ahi tuna steak, whole grain rice, bok choy

DAY 29

Breakfast: Red flannel hash

Snack: Half grapefruit, cottage cheese

Lunch: Ahi tuna salad

Snack: Kale chips

Dinner: Pulled tandoori chicken, roasted garlic carrots, kale chips

DAY 30

Breakfast: Smoked salmon eggs benedict

Snack: Poached pear

Lunch: Roasted chicken, mustard green salad with walnuts and raspberries

Snack: Faux-lafel with tzatziki sauce

Dinner: Pot roast with caramelized onions, creamy mashed sweet potatoes

Chapter 8. Life without Sugar

Life without sugar, or at least without refined and added sugars, can sound like a daunting task. In actuality it is simply claiming independence from unhealthy processed foods and refusing to sabotage your own body by pouring sugar in the gas tank, as it were.

When you choose to veer away from sugar, by necessity it removes almost all prepackaged foods and beverages. Cutting out sugar is an elegant solution to striving for a healthier lifestyle, period.

Embracing a sugar free lifestyle is akin to time traveling to simpler times, before sugar was shoved in our faces, down our throats, and into our homes by multitrillion dollar corporations.

Yes, sugar has always existed in one form or another, but the human body just isn't built to consume the quantities of sugar and the forms of sugar that are readily available.

Here is some food for thought: 100 years ago, obesity, cholesterol issues, heart disease, and type II diabetes were almost nonexistent. Compare that to now, where it is absolutely commonplace.

The American Psychological Foundation published a study which concluded that self-control is a limited resource which needs managing on a constant basis so it does not atrophy like a muscle that never gets exercised, or overwork it and burn it out.

The scientists conducting the study offer the advice to keep your limitations and boundaries at a happy medium. Don't bother with diets that ultimately make you feel worse than when you started.

Instead, save the self-control energy for the things that really holds the most meaning for you. Whether it is your career, love, traveling the world, or just who you strive to be in life, your natural appetite for surrounding yourself with things that are good for you will steadily reshape your world in beautiful light. This is true no matter what your worldview may be – you get out of it what you put into it.

When you choose to cut unhealthy foods from your healthy new life, you will be able to trust what your body wants more consistently.

Have an insatiable craving for a steak or feel like you could eat a whole turkey? You will be able to trust that your body needs protein, stat. Of course you won't eat the whole turkey. Because sugar is no longer running amok in your body, your body will be able to tell when you are full, and an hour later you will still feel satisfied instead of ravenous – like you always used to.

This feeling of being satisfied that you are adequately fed and no longer require sustenance for the time being is what will keep weight off in the long run, for the rest of your life in fact.

When you cut back on all of that unhealthy sugar, eventually you will come to a point where even milk tastes sweet. Like, really sweet. Milk's naturally occurring sugar, known as lactose, is actually a healthy sugar and one you are allowed to consume even in a strict sugar free lifestyle.

Fruit works much the same way, but there are rules involved there. It's better to focus on eating more of the low-glycemic fruits like raspberries and apples. A rough guide to eating fruit on a sugar free diet when in doubt is, the juicier the fruit is, the smaller amounts you should consume, as well as less frequently.

Once you rid all of that refined added sugar from your diet, you will notice the natural sweetness of certain foods you never in a million years would have considered sweet.

All in all, even something that you would have steered clear from in the past, say, broccoli, you would be able to taste the sweetness in and the flavor will be stronger as well. You will actually be able to taste your food!

You will notice so many changes once you cut sugar from life. If you're like most people, you've probably dreamed of one day attaining those sculpted abs or flat tummy.

A lifestyle that actively omits sugar enables you to achieve such a goal. Your dream body can actually be attainable (within reason, of course. A person who is naturally big boned will never be petite and be healthy. The same as someone who is rail thin will end up with a body builder's muscle definition).

It is possible to reach for the stars while still having your feet planted firmly on solid ground. The key is moderation. One thing a sugar free diet will teach you is that there is no need for all of the constant excess.

It feels amazing to actually be really hungry and to actually fill up on a tasty balanced meal. It may sound trivial, but the actuality is astounding. You will definitely become a more thankful individual.

One of the biggest challenges you may face after conquering the sugar addiction is probably going to be the convenience factor.

It used to be so easy to just grab something to eat on the go, but not so much once you commit to being sugar free. Gone are the days of just popping into a convenience store on your way to some place and picking up whatever prepackaged goodness caught your eye.

A lot of the times people shopping at convenient stores buy more than they need or even want, because they cannot make a decision as to what 'looks good'. The reason people may be unable to find what they're looking for is because it's just not there, even if you have a sweet tooth a mile wide.

Your body knows what it needs, and tries desperately to communicate these needs. Unfortunately, we are too busy shoving that pink coconut flavored marshmallow-y thing down our throats in a semi-successful attempt at tricking the body.

We tend to justify these behaviors in ways like, "I wasn't allowed to have that as a kid." It's pretty funny, but only because it is so true. You will find that you have to plan your meals a lot more and cook a lot more.

Another thing that you may find challenging is that when you may have those emotional roller coaster days of weaning yourself off of sugar, like any decent addict, you want the substance of your addiction all the more because it is comforting to you. It makes you feel good. You want it. You need it.

Many people have had this experience while overcoming their sugar addiction. It is completely normal and if it happens to you, you are not alone. There are many resources available to you online and probably in your community that you're not even aware of because you've never really viewed a high level of sugar intake as a sugar addiction.

If you're not exactly keen on hopping online to converse with people you will never see, about a problem you may not even be sure you have, or if an AA type meeting is just not in cards, it is recommended that you invite someone to do the sugar detox with you.

You don't necessarily have to be close to this person, but it would definitely help if you come within the same general proximity at least once a week. An important thing to remember is to just make it work for you.

Chapter 9.Tips on Staying Sugar Free

Once you've successfully completed the detox and made the decision to move forward with your newfound freedom from sugar, there are definitely a few solid tips on staying sugar free.

- Mentally prepare yourself for what lays ahead, both the positive and negative. It is so important to not worry; worrying defeats one of the hugest perks of being sugar free. Instead just realize that you may have ups and downs, and either way, it's going to pay off in a big way.

- Plan out your meals completely. Whether you scribble the meals and their recipes on a scrap piece of paper and stick it to the fridge or prefer to keep a file on your computer, just write them down in one way or another. This will be a big help in keeping you focused and prepared, and leave less room for a lapse.

- Say no. Say it out loud if you have to. This will strengthen your resolution immensely. The more times you say no, and are successful, the easier it will be next time.

- Do not, under any circumstances, ever have sugar in your house. Ever. Period. It would be like a crack head trying to go through recovery in a crack den. Don't do that to yourself.

- Research. There is quite a bit of material out there available to you 24 hours a day on this thing called the internet. Use it.

- Move it! Get out of your own way and get all physical and sweaty. Whatever exercise you prefer, make it work for you – and work hard. The natural endorphins your body creates from physical activity make you feel happy and make you want to repeat that happiness. This step is especially critical because you're removing something from your body that it thinks makes it feel good, and it's your job to replace it with something that actually is. Tough love!

- Take responsibility. It is important to pay attention to what you are eating. Maybe having a cheat day with sugar is not such a bright idea. If you've ever known anyone with an addiction, you know that the concept just doesn't work in the realm of addiction.

- Have fun with your sugar free self! You are on a great adventure! Move over, giant white whales, swashbuckling pirates, jungle boys, flying nannies, and cartoon princesses – make way for [your name here], who is rediscovering food; and for all intents and purposes, is the brand new owner of a new lease on life. There is genius in simplicity after all.

- Stock your cupboards and refrigerator to the brim with sugar free, easy to eat snacks. You will thank yourself. You will miss the convenience of sugar, and since we are used to overindulging, the muscle memory of constantly snacking will be in full force. Having a plethora of sugar free snacks at your fingertips may be the difference between a slip up and staying the course.

- Lend a hand. If you feel overwhelmed or underwhelmed or that roller coaster starts to become too much, it is human nature and way too easy to start feeling sorry for ourselves. Instead of wallowing in your sugary misery, lend a hand to your fellow human.

  If you're unaware of anyone who could use a random act of kindness and feel weird asking, go online. There are a plethora of volunteer opportunities out there. Many of which could really use the extra set of hands.

  Try your local food bank or other nonprofits. This will get your selfish 'me me me' brain to focus on 'hi, what can I do for you'. This will lend a lot of perspective and much needed objectivity when you may come across people who can't afford to feed their families or get to walk a puppy that is just the cutest fur ball you have ever seen. It works.

- Keep progress reports and know what you are up against. Usually by the fourth day or so, your sugar withdrawals will be at their strongest. It is difficult not to revert to a junkie mentality, making up ridiculous excuses to those who know your plight, as to why just one won't hurt.

  One bite, one scoop, just one. Well, as we all know, there is no such thing as just one. If you feel like you need it that badly, odds are you don't. Your rational brain right now thinks that this sounds dramatic, if not slightly hysterical.

  Keep that in mind. Make it a mantra. 'My rational brain knows that I do not need that disgusting sugar, it is hurting me. It is not good for me.' Or whatever you think will work for you. Just prepare yourself mentally for what may and most likely will, come.

It is equally important to equal that out with some resolute positive thinking. 'That will probably be difficult for me but I am strong and I will feel so proud when I overcome the sugar addiction.' You get the idea...or you will soon (wink, wink). You got this!

- Keep your mind engaged. Play chess or backgammon for the first time this decade. Kick back with a book or crossword. Play minesweeper. If you're a creative type, create! Build something. Groom your pet. Prep your meals for the next day.

Just as important as physical activity is mental activity. The more idle time your brain has, the more it will focus on the fact that it wants sugar. Right now. Now. How about now?

So, maybe refrain from binge watching your new favorite series every day. Maybe save the binge for a reward when you need it. It seems as though binge watching shows or movies is America's new favorite pastime. When most people binge watch, there is usually a plethora of snacks involved. So when you do need to watch for hours at a time, at least make sure you have plenty of those sugar free snacks close at hand.

Conclusion

Thank you again for buying this book!

I hope this book was able to help you on your journey into and through the sugar detox, as well as starting your exciting new sugar free lifestyle.

The next step is to put the recipes and meal plan into practice and make it work for you in the most efficient and personal way possible.

Finally, if you enjoyed this book, please take the time to share your thoughts and post a review on Amazon. I would sincerely appreciate it!

Thank you and the best of luck to you!